The Healing Mi
Apple Cider Vinegar &
Coconut Oil

Discover Natural Cures, Vibrant Health, Dramatic Weight Loss And More!

Table of Contents

Introduction

I want to thank you and congratulate you for downloading the book, "Apple Cider Vinegar and Coconut Oil".

This book contains proven steps and strategies on how to utilize apple cider vinegar and coconut oil in your daily health regimen. This book also gives you a list of health benefits of these super foods, individually and together. Real life transformations have also been listed out to give you an idea about how effective these ingredients are.

Unlike other books that give you just the theoretical side, this book gives you simple practical tips that you can make use of in your daily life. Apple cider vinegar and coconut oil are important ingredients in the health regiment of several celebrities. So, not only are they cheap, reliable and extremely effective, these two simple ingredients are your ticket to Hollywood Well-being.

This book is a result of extensive research on the two ingredients. I can vouch for several tips that have been provided in this book as I have tried them on myself and have found them extremely useful. These derivations from personal experiences ensure that everything that is listed in this book is tested to be safe and reliable. I do hope you have similar, if not better results with these tips using apple cider vinegar and coconut oil.

Thanks again for downloading this book, I hope you enjoy it

Chapter 1: Nature's most powerful health Supplements

For several centuries, natural products have been used as reliable health supplements and remedies. Before we got into prescribed medication and chemically created remedies, humans had no other option but to look at nature for solutions to several health problems. Needless to say, there have been ancient medical manuscripts that list out the uses and health benefits of these products. Two ingredients form an important part of oriental and western traditional remedies- apple cider vinegar and coconut oil.

Today, the health benefits of these miracle products of nature have been rediscovered. They have emerged as useful health tonics and have also made their way into the closets of several renowned celebrities. Before we get into the details of using apple cider vinegar and coconut oil in your own health regimen, let us first learn what these two super foods actually are. How are they derived? What do they contain? What makes them safe and reliable?

Apple Cider Vinegar

We all know that vinegar has been the main ingredient in several common recipes. From pickles to salads, we have seen the use of vinegar as a very useful preservative. In addition to that, it has also been used as a cleaning agent to make mirrors and metallic objects sparkle. Of course, it has been used as a folk remedy to help people relieve themselves of all possible ailments.

The contents of Apple Cider Vinegar are easy to guess. The name gives it all away. This is a pale, amber colored liquid that has been derived from cider or apples. To make apple cider vinegar, apples are crushed and squeezed until all the juices have been extracted. To this extract, bacteria and yeast is added to initiate the fermentation process. This fermentation is known as alcoholic fermentation as all the sugars in the apple extract are converted into alcohol.

Vinegar is chemically known as acetic acid. So the next step is to convert the fermented apple extract into vinegar. In this process, a strain of bacteria that forms acetic acid is used to convert the alcohol into acetic acid. It is this step that gives apple cider vinegar its trademark sour taste.

The unique taste of apple cider vinegar makes it a great ingredient for salad dressings, marinades, vinaigrettes and also chutneys.

Coconut Oil

A popular ingredient in oriental medicine, coconut oil has been consumed and applied externally for overall health benefits, for centuries. This natural extract from mature coconuts is a beauty and health package that is economical, easy to use and also free from side effects. The best part about coconut oil is that the shelf life is high and it can be stored for close to two years in its best condition.

You can get both edible and inedible coconut oils in stores. The edible form of coconut oil is usually refined, bleached and deodorized. Virgin coconut oil is considered the best as it is low in carbs and forms a great source of nutrition. Coconut oil that has been derived from copra as the starting product is usually unsuitable for consumption and can be applied externally only. So, if you are purchasing coconut oil, make sure you confirm that it is suitable for consumption to prevent avoidable health problems.

We will learn more about the types of apple cider vinegar and coconut oil in the following chapters so that you can make an informed decision when you decide to buy them.

Chapter 2: Types of ACV and Coconut Oil

Depending upon the process of manufacturing, you can obtain several types of coconut oil and apple cider vinegar. Each type has different benefits and functions. It is necessary for you to know what types are available so that you can decide how to use them. You see, some forms of apple cider vinegar and coconut oil can be used only for external application. Consumption of these types can be hazardous to your health. So, if you are considering including apple cider vinegar and coconut oil in your health routine, this chapter must be read with very close attention.

Types of Apple Cider Vinegar

Apple cider vinegar as we know now is a fermented product derived from apples. There are basically two types of apple cider vinegar that are found in stores:

Raw Apple Cider Vinegar

This is the natural form of apple cider vinegar. It is known for its strong flavor that works beautifully with different kinds of salads and pickles. Of course, the health benefits of raw apple cider vinegar are also many. You will be able to identify raw apple cider vinegar with its color and texture. It is a bright, amber colored liquid. It has a cloudy appearance because it contains "mother of vinegar"

Mother of vinegar is a stringy substance that is naturally formed when the apple extracts are fermented. This is gelatinous in texture and is considered to be very good for your health as it contains all the 'good bacteria' and the raw enzymes. This type of apple cider vinegar, although very useful, is slightly difficult to store. You must maintain recommended conditions and also the pH balance of the tonic to ensure that there is not bacterial growth in it.

Pasteurized Apple Cider Vinegar

Pasteurization is a type of treatment that is given to foods to make them suitable for consumption. The main objective of pasteurization is to destroy certain strains of microorganisms that can be very harmful to general health. In this process, the apple cider vinegar is exposed to high temperatures in which the undesirable microorganisms cannot flourish.

Pasteurized apple cider vinegar is clear in its appearance. This is because the "mother of vinegar" is removed to make give it a sparkling clean appearance. Several health experts argue that this method removes the natural goodness of apple cider vinegar which forms the basis of all the health treatments.

However, storage is not a problem with pasteurized apple cider vinegar as the chances of bacterial growth are much lower. This clear appearance is also more appealing to consumers and is therefore promoted by most manufacturers. The only common thing between the two kinds of apple cider vinegar is that the core element that gives them a characteristic taste and odor is the acetic acid. However, there are several reasons why you must choose organic apple cider vinegar over the pasteurized variety. We will discuss this in detail in the following chapters so that you are able to get the exact distinction and hence, understand the advantages of the organic variety.

Types of Coconut Oil

Coconut Oil is available in several forms that can be used for cooking, medicinal purposes and also for external application. There are four types of coconut oil that are commonly found in all the supermarkets and food stores:

Refined Coconut Oil

Coconut oil that is used for commercial purposes is usually made from copra. Copra is obtained by drying up the meat of a mature coconut. Usually, copra is made using methods like kiln drying, sun drying and smoke drying. Sometimes, the meat dries up naturally when in the tree due to certain weather conditions. This type of coconut oil that is derived from copra is not suitable for edible uses unless it is completely refined. The reason for refining coconut oil is actually the unhygienic methods that are usually adopted to make copra.

In order to make refined coconut oil, the extracts go through several processes. The first step is deodorizing the oil using steam. Next it is passed through several bleaching clays to remove any traces of impurities. The last stage is to make sure that the coconut oil lasts long enough. This is achieved by removing all the free fatty acids using sodium hydroxide. Earlier, coconut oil was extracted using mechanical methods. However, today, coconut oil is extracted using chemical solvents to ensure that the amount of oil extracted is higher. Modern methods of extraction ensure that there is no wastage of the oils contained in the copra.

Hydrogenated Coconut Oil

In most cases, the coconut oil that is refined, bleached and deodorized is hydrogenated fully or completely. This practice is common in tropical areas as the melting point of coconut oil is about 76 degrees F. The coconut oil retains its natural solid state in colder conditions. One common issue with coconut oil is the hydrogenation process itself. Coconut oil contains very little unsaturated oil which makes it hard to hydrogenate. Once it is hydrogenated, however, it contains traces of trans-fatty acids.

As a result, several authorities like the FDA are considering banning hydrogenated coconut oil. It is mandatory for the manufacturers of hydrogenated coconut oils to provide details of the trans-fats. So, instead of making just the hydrogenated coconut oils available, there are several candy bars and other tropical products that use hydrogenated coconut oil as one of the ingredients. This is done usually when they want to ensure that the coconut oil in the product does not melt. However, several European countries have banned hydrogenated coconut oil altogether.

Liquid Coconut Oil

This is a unique inclusion in the market that has been promoted widely as exclusive 'cooking oil'. The interesting thing about this type of coconut oil is that it never turns into fat. Therefore it remains in its liquid form in almost all temperatures including when it is kept in the refrigerator. Because of this property, there have been several debates if it is, in fact, a pure form of coconut oil or not.

The term "fat" is used with reference to coconut oil only when it gets solidified. In colder regions this is a common phenomenon. However, in tropical countries where coconut oil is actually grown, this is not an issue as the temperature in these areas is always maintained above 70 degrees Fahrenheit. Under these conditions, the coconut oil remains in its liquid form.

Liquid coconut oil is definitely not a natural product. It is manufactured by removing some fatty acids that are commonly found in coconut oil. Usually, using the fractioning method, the saturated fatty acids are removed from the coconut oil as they are the ones that attain the solid form when the oil is exposed to colder temperatures.

One of the most predominant fatty acids of coconut oil, lauric acid, is extracted in the manufacturing process of liquid coconut oil. This fatty acid has been researched about extensively and has been linked with several health benefits. All the other fatty acids that have high melting points are also removed to make sure that this product remains in its liquid form. Now, the most commonly asked question about liquid coconut oil is whether it is suitable for any health related use.

Of course, the nutritional value of this oil is severely reduced. However, it is used for application on the skin as it is more easily and readily absorbed than other forms of coconut oil.

Virgin Coconut Oil

This is the most beneficial and, perhaps, the most widely used form of coconut oil. Unlike olive oil which has certain set standards for "virgin" and "extra virgin" oils, coconut oil does not really have any industry standards. There are several brands of virgin and extra virgin coconut oils that are available in the market today. What forms the basis of virgin coconut oil is the manufacturing process.

The most common way of extracting coconut oil is by drying the meat of the coconut using kiln drying or smoke drying methods. Then this dried copra is pressed out to release the oils. The expeller-pressing method is used in the industrial manufacturing process. Virgin coconut oil is usually found in tropical countries as they have well- established methods of producing copra. This allows them to extract the oils and sell them.

The wet milling process is also used to extract virgin coconut oil. In this method, coconut milk is extracted from the coconut meat first. The oil and the water is then separated to produce coconut oil using a centrifuge.

Virgin coconut oil is used in several medicinal preparations. It is especially useful for external application as it is easily absorbed by the skin and the hair.

Once you are sure of how you want to use apple cider vinegar and coconut oil, you can decide what variety you want to buy. For you to choose the most practical application of these products, read the following chapters.

Chapter 3: Health Benefits

Both coconut oil and Apple Cider Vinegar have been proven to be extremely useful in promoting health and general well being. There is also ample research available to help us understand the logical reasoning behind the benefits of these products. Here is a list of health benefits that will tell you what you can expect from apple cider vinegar and coconut oil.

Apple Cider Vinegar

Socrates made one of the earliest references to the benefits of using apple cider vinegar in curing health related issues. However, this product received predominance as an effective health tonic in recent years, especially in the middle of the twentieth century. It was during this age that several books were published about the health benefits of apple cider vinegar along with scientific evidence that supported these claims.

In the year 1958, a book titled "Folk Medicine: A Vermont Doctor's Guide to Good Health" was published by an author named D.C Jarvis, M.D. Dr. Jarvis who was a noted doctor from Vermont reported the Apple Cider Vinegar has the ability to cure all ailments. This product had an unusually high level of potassium and was, hence, very effective when combined with other natural products like honey. It was after the publication of this book that the medicinal uses of apple cider vinegar became well known.

Apple cider vinegar has been used widely in the remedies for:

Type 2 Diabetes

The main ingredient of apple cider vinegar is acetic acid. This makes it very acidic in nature. It is this property of apple cider vinegar that has been found extremely useful in curing type 2 and type 1 diabetes. The main reason why apple cider vinegar is useful in curing diabetes is that it has the ability to lower the level of glucose in the blood.

The most common disorders related to blood sugar are due to changes in the diet and the change caused by different foods in the level of blood sugar in the body. This influence of foods on the blood sugar level is measured using a term called the glycemic index of the food. Foods like potato, processed grains and even sugar have a high glycemic index which results in an increase in the sugar levels of the blood. On the other hand low glycemic index foods like beans and grains create less drastic changes in the blood sugar levels.

It is possible to keep the blood sugar level stable if the amount of consumption of high GI food is controlled. Because of the acidic property of apple cider vinegar, it plays a significant role in the reduction of the glycemic index of foods. Basically, it is able to reduce the speed at which the carbohydrates present in these foods are converted into glucose.

The main function of apple cider vinegar is to soak up all the bicarbonates that are present in the lower intestine. Without this bicarbonate, the rate of absorption of carbohydrates comes down drastically. Health experts refer to this phenomenon as "delayed gastric emptying". Logically, slower absorption of sugars results in reduced blood sugar levels. This phenomenon is especially beneficial to people with type 2 diabetes as they rely upon reduced rate of glucose consumption to maintain homeostasis in their bodies.

Several studies have been conducted to understand the effect of apple cider vinegar on diabetic individuals. One such study that was published in the journal of the American Diabetes association stated that Insulin sensitivity to a meal with high carbohydrate content was improved to a large extent in people with Type 2 diabetes. This condition is usually characterized by insulin resistance. In this study, the subjects were divided into three groups- diabetic, pre diabetics and people with normal blood sugar levels.

Each group was given 2 two table spoons of apple cider vinegar before two meals each day. It was observed that the group in the pre diabetic stage showed maximum results when they consumed apple cider vinegar. The level of blood sugar dropped by 50% in this group. The next group consisted of individuals who had already been diagnosed with diabetes. In this group, the blood sugar level improved by 25%. The conclusion that was drawn from this study was that apple cider vinegar had the same effect on individuals as metformin, as that of a drug prescribed to treat type 2 diabetes.

Even in healthy individuals, the consumption of apple cider vinegar has very interesting effects. It is known to reduce the postprandial blood sugar levels by almost 20%. Another research conducted in the Department of Nutrition at the Ahvaz Jundishapour University in Iran showed that with just four weeks of administering Apple cider vinegar in diabetic individuals, the level of bad cholesterol or LDL cholesterol was significantly reduced. In the other hand, the level of good cholesterol or HDL was increased significantly.

With these studies, it becomes clear that Apple Cider Vinegar is pivotal in helping diabetic individuals manage their condition. Of course, there is no clarity on how apple cider vinegar actually works in accomplishing this. Nevertheless, apple cider vinegar has been tested and used successfully in reducing the blood sugar levels in individuals suffering from diabetes.

Also, the effects of Apple Cider Vinegar are similar to prescribed medicines that have been used to treat type 1 and type 2 diabetes. From this, it becomes clear that using a natural substitute to control a certain condition is better than using chemically prepared drugs.

Apple cider vinegar is a definite precautionary measure against diabetes. Therefore, it is recommended that even health individuals must consume apple cider vinegar on a regular basis to control the possibility of acquiring this condition.

In case you have already been diagnosed with type 1 or type 2 diabetes, it is recommended that you consult your doctor before using apple cider vinegar. If you are in the pre-diabetic stage, however, this is the best remedy to help control the chances of a full blown condition of diabetes.

Apple Cider Vinegar and Acid Reflux

Acid reflux is a common digestive disorder. It is known to create a lot of uneasiness and discomfort. Now, what exactly is acid reflux?

The entrance to our stomach is controlled by a valve that is called the lower esophageal valve. This is a ring of muscles that open and close to allow the food into the stomach and to make sure that it remains there. This makes sure that all the food and the digestive enzymes that are produced remain within the stomach. Sometimes, however, the valve fails to close completely or might open often to allow the acids to go up the esophagus. This is what we often describe as heart burn or acid reflux.

This condition can be severely painful as it is accompanied by a burning sensation in the chest. Sometimes this condition is only temporary. It might be caused by lying down after a heavy meal and also indulging in midnight snacking. However, it can also be a recognized disease if it occurs more than twice a week. It is very common in people who are obese or overweight. It is also very common in people who are addicted to certain substances of beverages.

This condition is also known as gastro esophageal reflux disease. Another condition that occurs with this disease is hiatal hernia. In this condition the lower esophageal valve and the stomach move higher than the diaphragm. In this case, the diaphragm is unable to keep the acid within our stomach and hence worsens the condition.

Apple cider vinegar is a very common remedy for acid reflux and has been used for several decades to serve this purpose. What is bizarre or worth some thought is that fact that apple cider vinegar itself is highly acidic. So, how is it possible that it controls acid reflux and its symptoms? Also, acidic foods are never recommended for people with acid reflux? So, how is it that apple cider vinegar made the cut to the list of recommended acid reflux remedies? There are several theories that support this bizarre medical remedy. However, the actual reason for this choice of medication is still not known.

The only possible explanation for this is that apples and apple cider vinegar contain common enzymes. After all, apple cider vinegar is just a fermented form of apples. Now, apples have been recommended as a suitable remedy for acid reflux. This is possible because apples are able to protect our intestines and hence reduce the chances of acid reflux. Apple cider vinegar is very useful in reducing the pH levels of our blood. This, in turn, helps the intestine fight harmful bacteria and fungi that cause acid reflux in many cases. Apple cider vinegar also contains proven antimicrobial properties that help maintain intestinal health. When the health of the intestine is maintained, the possibility of acid reflux is reduced to a large extent. However, this just comes across as a preventive measure.

Apple Cider Vinegar, on the other hand, is useful even when you are already suffering from acid reflux. According to the Maryland Medical centre, taking two teaspoons of apple cider vinegar with warm water has the ability to prevent food poisoning and can also control the symptoms of acid reflux.

There are some theories that state the possible ways in which apple cider vinegar reacts in our body to produce the desired out come. The first theory is that apple cider vinegar has a natural acidic property that is useful in breaking down fats easily. This is very useful in speeding up the process of digestion. Digestion is also eased to reduce the symptoms of acid reflux.

Other theories suggest that the production of acids in the stomach is regulated with the help of apple cider vinegar. The acetic acid in the apple cider vinegar acts as a buffer for the level of acidity in the stomach. This is because acetic acid is not as strong as the hydrochloric acid that is produced in the stomach. This acts as a balancing agent and hence controls the acidity in our stomach.

While these are only possibilities and theories, the only thing that we know for sure is that apple cider vinegar is highly useful in providing relief from acid reflux. When this product is consumed in its organic form, especially, the benefits are many. Because of the immediate relief and the long term benefits, apple cider vinegar has been voted as the most reliable natural remedy for acid reflux.

Apple Cider Vinegar and Weight Loss

Apple cider vinegar is most often used for its ability to cut down fats and help us drastically reduce weight. For this reason, apple cider vinegar has actually found its way into several ancient remedies to maintain physical health.

Today we consume apple cider vinegar in the form of salads and even tablets to aid weight loss. With the current need to look good all the time and to have the most desired hour-glass figure, several celebrities and health experts have turned to the best and most natural weight loss remedy, apple cider vinegar. This ingredient, when made a part of our regular diet, has the ability to cut down weight, make us feel more energetic and just improve our overall well being.

The best part is that there are no severe side effects. This product is completely natural and safe and is therefore the best weight loss solution available to us today.

Ancient recipes suggest that apple cider vinegar has the ability to reduce appetite and food cravings when consumed in right quantities. Metabolism is also stimulated when you consume apple cider vinegar. This is one of the most important requirements for anyone who is currently on the route to losing weight.

Weight loss is also significantly accelerated by apple cider vinegar because it has the ability to regulate the blood sugar levels in our body. This helps suppress hunger and therefore control your diet effectively.

Studies have been conducted to understand the relationship between weight loss and apple cider vinegar consumption. In 2009, a study conducted in Japan showed a significant effect on obese individuals when apple cider vinegar was administered to them on a regular basis. These individuals were given only 30 ml of vinegar each day. This caused a significant decrease in their weight as well as their appetite. This study revealed that vinegar intake has a lot of positive effects on body fat mass maintenance and also body weigh regulation. This is because of acetic acid that is useful in reducing the accumulation of fat in the body.

Including apple cider vinegar in your diet is recommended if you are looking at a natural and effective weight loss regimen. Apple cider vinegar has the ability to increase you metabolism and, hence, improve your chances of losing weight. Studies related to apple cider vinegar and weight loss also suggest that it is highly beneficial in maintaining the sugar balance in the body. The glycemic index of certain foods is reduced when apple cider vinegar is consumed. This property helps spike weight loss.

Apple cider vinegar also has the ability to control conditions like candida. This is a fungal infection that causes cravings for sugars and carbohydrates. This contributes to weight gain and is significantly controlled by using apple cider vinegar that has well known anti fungal properties.

The consumption of apple cider vinegar has another important result which is detoxification. The apple cider vinegar detox is one of the most significant fitness remedies in the world today. Since apple cider vinegar is extremely acidic in nature, it has the ability to boost digestion. In addition

These enzymes are very useful and form the basis of all the health benefits of apple vinegar cider. The process version is no doubt clear and more pleasant looking. However the nutritional benefits and other health benefits of this form of apple vinegar cider are fewer.

Even in case of coconut oil it is recommended that we only opt for virgin coconut oil which the purest and most natural form available. Undoubtedly colder countries may opt for the versions like liquid coconut oil in order to ensure that it doesn't harden in cold conditions. This variety of coconut is treated heavily and is stripped of the fatty acids which form the basis of the healing abilities of coconut oil.

There have been several debates about the safety and advantages of using organic products. However research today shows that we have no other choice but to go the organic way. In process foods and natural products several chemicals are used which render these otherwise useful products quite harmful. For instance processed apple vinegar cider or coconut oil can cause a lot of irritation and discomfort when used regularly. The organic product on the other hand is safe and can even be recommended for children.

Using Organic products can also be your way of contributing to the environment. Since these foods are grown without chemicals that are harmful to the environment they ensure that our planet does not deteriorate further. Using organic manures and pesticides make the soil richer. These plants require lesser water and hence play a pivotal role in water conservation.

Organic foods are best for consumption. These foods retain all the natural flavors that are most often missing in the processed versions. Obviously these foods taste better. Research shows that apple vinegar cider and coconut oil have maximum mineral salts in their organic forms. As a result the health benefits of these products are also greater.

I personally recommend the use of organic products if you have children and pets at home you might want to switch to an organic way of life altogether. So in case these foods are accidentally consumed by them there are no adverse effects on their health. I have tried organic apple vinegar cider and coconut oil and seen amazing results.

In addition to that, the intestine is also cleansed to remove bacteria and fungi that cause retention of fats causing weight gain. Because of its high acetic acid content, apple cider vinegar also has the ability to break down fatty acids in foods, making them easy to assimilate. So, it is recommended that you consume apple cider vinegar in recommended doses on a regular basis.

However, it is wrong to assume that apple cider vinegar is a magic bullet for weight loss. It is only a catalyst that aids your weight loss program. In order to have visible results, the consumption of apple cider vinegar must be accompanied by a good diet plan and a regular exercise routine. While apple cider vinegar is useful in weight loss, it cannot be used as the only component for a weight loss program.

Other health benefits of Apple Cider Vinegar

While the above mentioned benefits of apple cider vinegar are the most important and the most well known health benefits of the product, there are many more benefits of consuming apple cider vinegar on a regular basis. They include:

• **A Great Mouth Freshener:** There are many who swear by the ability of apple cider vinegar to reduce bad breath. All you need to do is mix some apple cider vinegar, mix it with some water and gargle it just as you would any other commercial mouth freshener. Because of its acidic property, apple cider vinegar not only reduces bad odor but also helps whiten teeth.

- **Remedy for Diarrhea:** Apple Cider vinegar is a very popular folk remedy for diarrhea. It is useful in getting rid of any bacterial infection in the intestines. The antibiotic properties of apple cider vinegar also calm muscle spasms in the intestines. All you need to do is mix some apple cider vinegar in water and consume it for best results.

- **The perfect Hiccups solution:** There are so many things that we try when we get hiccups, we hopelessly try to scare our selves, drink gallons and gallons of water, hold our breath and even eat peanut butter. Sometimes, they work. Most often, they don't. If you are looking for a remedy that can curb an uncontrollable round of hiccups, all you need to do is consume a teaspoon of apple cider vinegar. It will just reduce your hiccups within minutes.

- **The perfect sore throat remedy:** When you consume apple cider vinegar, you might have noticed a certain burning sensation that goes straight down till your tummy. This effect is rather soothing when you are suffering with a sore throat. The antibacterial property of apple cider vinegar is perfect to fight the infections that are usually the cause for a sore throat.

- **Get rid of the itch:** Have you ever been bugged by pesky mosquitoes that leave your skin feeling itchy and painful. Of course, mosquito bites are also famous for leaving horrible blisters and rashes that are not desirable at all. In such cases, all you need to do is take a swab of cotton, dip it in some apple cider vinegar and rub it on the affected area.

- **Manage blood pressure and cholesterol:** Studies have shown that consuming apple cider vinegar on a regular basis can help reduce the cholesterol levels in the blood significantly. It also lowers blood pressure and helps you keep your heart healthy and happy.

This chapter only covers the medical uses of apple cider vinegar. If we were to delve into the beauty benefits of apple cider vinegar, you would be astonished at how amazing this everyday household product actually is. And, you will wonder why you never tried it before!

Health benefits of Coconut Oil

Organic Coconut Oil is one of the healthiest oil that is in use. The number of health benefits of using coconut oil is countless. All the benefits are not mere assumptions but are also backed by extensive research. According to doctors it should be a part of your every day nutrition plan. Dr Mark Atkinson who gave the world one of the most nutritious and healthy diet plans also vouches for the health benefits of this miraculous natural extract.

For over 4000 years man has used coconut oil as a part of his nutritional plan and also medicinal remedies. There are several documents that support the use of coconut oil as food and also in pharmaceuticals. The positive thing all these records is that the results have always been good with very few cases of side effects and negative results. It has been mostly used in oriental medicine and countries like Africa and Southern America.

The use of coconut oil has been respected by all these cultures and also has been given spiritual connotations. In Sanskrit documents of Ayurvedic medicine which were made as early as 1500 BC, it has been stated that Coconut Oil heals the min d body and the spirit. Several European explorers including the likes of Captain Cook have written elaborately about the beauty of people across the pacific that made use of coconut oil in their daily lives.

During the Second World War coconut oil that was derived from young green coconut was actually used as a substitute for saline drips. It was influential in saving the lives of several soldiers during the war. Centuries later, coconut oil is still being recommended as one of the primary benefactors in our health and well being.

Coconut Oil and Diabetes

In the United States alone almost 8.3% of the population is affected with diabetes. This includes 25.8 million children. Every ten years the number of people becoming diabetic is doubling. As a result several pharmaceutical companies have started capitalizing on this epidemic by merely producing drugs that are able to control the condition but are not able to fight it by going to the underlying causes. In addition to that these drugs also have several side effects. Recently a very popular diabetic drug was pulled out of the market when studies showed that the consumption of this drug actually increased the risk of heart attack in diabetic patients. When we hear about such fraudulent companies and such irresponsible products being released into the market it questions our sense of well being.

It makes us wonder if we should look at natural and safer remedies for such ailments. Luckily for us nature is abundant with solutions to all our maladies, coconut oil being on the top of this list. Today mainstream media is making people aware that the treatment of diabetes lies mainly in our lifestyle and cannot be merely reversed with the use of drugs. This is something that the practitioners of alternative medicine have been preaching for several years.

Several diabetic individuals have started replacing vegetable oils with coconut oil in their cooking. Within a few months of this small change they have seen dramatic results when they checked their blood sugar levels. The levels have been stabilized and fluctuations have reduced considerably. Recommended diets for individuals who are diabetic include restricting carbohydrates, sugars and alcohol from their diet while decreasing the consumption of protein and saturated fats.

Coconut oil is the perfect replacement for polyunsaturated fats like soya bean oil and corn oil. The saturated fatty acids in coconut oil help reduce our cravings for refined carbohydrates. This in turn is useful in promoting insulin sensitivity.

In the year 1998 a research was conducted amongst groups of individuals in the Indian sub continent. Indians who have been traditionally using fats like coconut oil and ghee for cooking have turned to sun flower oils and other vegetable oils. This resulted in increase of the number of diabetics at an alarming rate. Similar results have also been found in other South Pacific Island Countries who have turned to modern processed foods that include the use of polyunsaturated fatty acids instead of their traditional coconut oil rich diet.

In 2009 Dr Nigel Turner conducted a study in Australia. His research demonstrated that coconut oil increases the ability of cells to respond to insulin. In other words it aids insulin sensitivity. Coconut oil that consists of medium chain fatty acids also prevents the accumulation of fats in our body. This is quite unlike refined oils that have long chains of fatty acids that are difficult to assimilate. These findings are important for two reasons. First they demonstrate the benefit of coconut oil in controlling diabetes. Second they highlight the benefits of coconut oil in preventing morbid obesity which is the prime contributing factor for the increase in the rate of diabetic individuals.

Type 2 diabetes is no doubt a lifestyle related problem. However Type 1 diabetes is caused by our body inability to produce insulin. The good news is that coconut oil has shown positive results in controlling Type 1 diabetes as well.

In 2009 a study conducted on the influence of coconut oil in Type 1 diabetes showed that the positive results were because of an improvement in the brain function. The conclusion of this study stated that the medium chain fatty acids in coconut oil had therapeutic results on the brain and were useful in preserving brain function. This improves the function of endocrine glands that are responsible for production of insulin. Several neurological disorders can also be controlled using coconut oil on a regular basis.

With these studies and research in place there is hope that we will be able to get over our dependency on chemically produced drugs and will be able to adopt natural remedies. These extracts from nature also have other positive results on our well being. So with these products being easily available we can hope for a population that is not only healthier but happier as well.

As our systems get used to these natural vitamins we will see that our internal well being is reflected externally as well .However these routines require lots of patience and faith that the results will be as we desire.

Coconut oil and weight loss

Seven individuals who have switched to virgin coconut oil have stated that it is influential in keeping the energy levels up. In comparison to other healthy oils the inclusion of coconut oil in the diet made all the difference. The reason for weight loss have been stated as increase energy levels, reduced need to consume carbohydrates and sweets and the feeling of being full and satisfied after every meal. The first step at appreciating the benefits of coconut oil is understanding that low fat diets are not the key to steady and healthy weight loss. We have all been told that the only way to lose weight is cutting back on the fat we consume. In fact many dietitians recommend this as the only way out. There are several companies that have backed these things because they manufacture low fat products.

The US Centre for disease control has revealed that the increase in obesity was noted only in the last 20 years. The rates are high even today and obesity is almost an epidemic.

In just 2 years the prevalence of obesity in the United States increased by 5% in some states and by a shocking 10% in others.

In one of his statements Tommy G Thompson, the Secretary of Health and Human Services stated that this profound increase in the number of obese people has led to severe health implications. Obese people are at the risk of diabetes, heart diseases, strokes and even some forms of Cancer.

Even after 10 years the situation has not really improved but has actually become worse. This means that low fat diets have not really helped in weight loss. After all, almost two thirds of adults in the U S have been classified as overweight. Many of them are already on torturous diet plans that recommend avoiding any fat consumption in their diet.

Before we shun fats we need to understand that they have been a part of our nutrition for centuries now. Until the 1940s only eggs, butter, nuts, animal fats were classified as high fats. Today almost every food falls in that category. In fact these high fat foods were also considered to be healthy at one point. Statistics show that even after drastically reducing the consumption of these fats in the modern diet no health problems have been resolved and obesity rates are only increasing. Now we are left with only one choice considering the possibility of a hypothesis that is contrary to modern dietary beliefs. This is possible only when we explore the food habits of traditional societies and also our forefathers. These people have been consuming the same kind of food for centuries and have managed to remain healthy and even slim. The fats that are a part of their diet were actually rich in saturated fatty acids. In many tropical areas palm oil and coconut oil have been consumed traditionally.

Of these two kinds of oils coconut oil has some rather unique properties. It consists of medium chain of fatty acids that are similar to the fats found in breast milk. Research shows that this property aids in metabolism and therefore leads to weight loss. In comparison to other plant based oils that contain long chain of fatty acids, coconut oil is a much better option for consumption. These long chains are usually retained in the body in the form of fats. On the other hand the medium chain fatty acids found in coconut oil are utilized to create energy. They burn very quickly in our body and are not retained.

Medium chain fatty acids promote a process called thermogenesis. This is the body's ability to metabolize the foods that are consumed to produce energy. A study conducted in Japan showed that foods rich in medium chain fatty acids have the property of increasing thermogenesis as their metabolized almost as soon as they are consumed. To prove this they conducted a study on two groups of animals. The group that was given vegetable oils produced meat that was fatty. On the other hand animals that were given coconut oil provided lean meat.

This only goes to show that coconut oil is a great substitute in our diet. However they have been testimonies of people who have stated that coconut oil did not really help lose any weight. At this point I would like to remind my readers that there is no short cut to weight loss. Foods like coconut oil only speed up the process but must be accompanied by exercise and healthy eating habits to see results.

Coconut oil and immunity

Our immune system plays a most important role in our survival. This is our body's defense mechanism against several micro organisms that we come in contact with almost every second. It is our job to make sure that we maintain our immune system by providing it with the right amount of nutrition. If you are looking at natural remedies to help you develop a dynamic and robust immune system there is no better option than coconut oil.

In comparison to all fats and oils that constitute our diet coconut oil has the highest amount of immune boosting fatty acids. The main constituent of coconut oil called Lauric acid is converted into a very powerful antiviral anti fungal and antibiotic agent known as Monlaurin. Again this molecule is very similar to the constituent found in the breast milk of the mother which provides infants with immunity in their delicate years. There are several man-made immune boosters that are available. However Lauric acid is the safest option. It is more powerful and is able to destroy many harmful micro organisms without causing harm to the cells present in our body. When applied topically coconut oil enhances tissue repair and prepares the first step of immunity which is our skin. Caprylic acid is a powerful antifungal agent that is found in coconut oil. As a result using coconut oil regularly helps heal cuts, rashes and dry skin. When consumed internally, these anti microbial properties benefit the entire body and help fight diseases effectively.

Most diseases that we contract are either due to bacteria or virus. Since coconut oil consists of so many anti-viral and anti bacterial properties you can be assured that your body will be safe from diseases all year long. There are several studies that promote the use of coconut oil in boosting immunity. One study conducted on the harmful bacteria found near our mouth showed that coconut oil is more powerful than we believe. In extension to this research several manufacturers are trying to understand if the inclusion of coconut oil and its compounds in oral health care products especially toothpastes will have any effect on our overall well being. After all it has been studied that oral health is one of the most important contributors to a healthy body. Studies have also shown that mortality and oral health are actually related. This is because having poor health leads to an increase in harmful bacteria all over the body as the mouth forms the first point of entry for these harmful microbes. If left unattended these bacteria have the potential to harm our immune system and cause a lot of damage. Coconut oil decreases the population of these bacteria and therefore able to promote good health. The metabolic properties of coconut oil are also useful in healing individuals who might be fatigued or unwell. Consuming coconut oil provides a much needed burst of energy for these individuals. Coconut oil is easily absorbed by all our cells therefore is particularly useful to people who are unable to consume proper meals.

Coconut oil is considered an overall health food and a natural healer. It is recommended that every individual must consume at least 24 grams of coconut oil every day in order to improve its protective function. This means, on an average one must consume at least 3.5 tablespoons of coconut oil every day. This amount is equivalent to consuming almost an entire coconut in a day.

Coconut oil is not just an extract but is a complete food by itself. So you may consider using it in snacks, salads and smoothies and other forms of foods. Immunity is not as simple as consuming one food that has the ability to boost it. If you are leading an unhealthy life that includes several trans-fats, processed foods and unhealthy habits all the coconut oil in the world will not make a difference. Coconut oil has dramatic effects on health only when it is added to the diet of a person who is already following a healthy way of life.

Other health benefits of Coconut oil

The health benefits stated above are among the most well known health benefits of coconut oil. However there are many constituents in coconut oil that can be well wisher to our health in several ways. Some additional health benefits of coconut oil are:

Reduction of seizures-Coconut oil is also known as a Ketogenic. This means that coconut oil is high in fats but low in carbohydrates. One of the most important therapeutic applications of coconut oil is treating epilepsy that is resistant to drugs. When the number of Ketone bodies in the blood increase there is a dramatic decrease in the number of seizures experienced by people with epilepsy.

The exact reason for this effect is not known. However even people who have not had any relief from epilepsy after using recommended drugs have noticed benefits of coconut oil in controlling the condition. The only theory available states that the medium chain fatty acids are converted to Ketone in the body to yield desirable results.

Controlling blood cholesterol level-Most of us refrain from consuming coconut oil because we believe that the saturated fatty acids present in it will increase level of cholesterol. However quite contrary to these beliefs there is no change in the blood lipid profile because of coconut oil. In fact in a study conducted on 40 women it was noted that coconut oil reduced the total cholesterol level of the blood. Now there are two types of cholesterol, HDL cholesterol or good cholesterol and LDL Cholesterol or the bad cholesterol. This study revealed that HDL Cholesterol in the blood increased while LDL Cholesterol decreased considerably. This made the body's anti oxidant status high and also aided in blood coagulation. This also improved heart health and reduced the risks of acquiring heart diseases over a period of time.

Boosts Brain Function-Across the world Alzheimer's disease is the main cause for Dementia in elders. In this condition the brain loses its ability to metabolize glucose to produce energy in certain parts. Therefore this region of the brain is unable to function naturally and requires an alternate source of energy to improve the condition of the cells. Several researchers have speculated that this alternate source of energy can be produced by Ketone bodies. In 2006 a study conducted on patients with milder forms of the condition showed that brain functions improve significantly when coconut oil is consumed regularly. This is because the medium chain fatty acids provide a source of alternate energy in the form of Ketone bodies. As a result the symptoms of Alzheimer's disease are reduced and coconut oil is used as a proven therapeutic measure against the condition.

Curbs Hunger-When you include coconut oil in your meals you will notice that your hunger level decreases. This phenomenon is also related to the production of Ketone bodies upon the breakdown of the medium fatty acids. When you consume coconut oil the consumption of calories reduces significantly. When you consume coconut oil in one meal you will notice that the size and portion of the next meal reduces to a large extent. Because of this you are also able to keep a check on your weight.

So you see products that are as simple as coconut oil and Apple Cider Vinegar can have profound health benefits. Several individuals have also used them successfully in creating home remedies for several cosmetic issues. The next chapter in detail the beauty benefits of Apple Cider Vinegar and coconut oil.

Chapter 4: Beauty Secrets Revealed

One aspect of healthcare that we are highly conscious of is our beauty regimen. This is one area where we cannot take any risk as defects are too obvious and sometimes disastrous to our psychological well being. Many celebrities endorse the use of coconut oil and Apple Cider Vinegar to reap excellent benefits. These methods have been used for centuries and are therefore highly reliable. The side effects are lesser and therefore we can use these methods without worrying too much.

Apple Cider Vinegar for the hair

Apple Cider Vinegar is a great treatment for the hair. Although it might seem like a rather unconventional method Apple Cider Vinegar when mixed with other natural ingredients like Greek Yogurt and Honey can transform the appearance of your hair. Here are a few ways in which you can use Apple Cider Vinegar for your hair.

1.   **As a Hair Conditioner**- If you are struggling with frizzy and unmanageable hair what you need is a good conditioner. Apple Cider Vinegar should be rubbed gently into the scalp and along the length of your hair with a dash of

baking soda. This combination nourishes and conditions hair leaving it soft, smooth and supple.

2.   **Increasing Porosity of the Hair**- Our hair maintains its natural sheen because of its ability to hold moisture within it. This characteristic of the hair is known as porosity.   When hair fails to absorb moisture and keep it locked within itself it causes a very brittle hair shaft. As a result hair becomes lifeless and it is prone to breakage. Using Apple Cider Vinegar on the hair can improve porosity. This is because the acidity of Apple Cider Vinegar seals the cuticle of the hair and hence allows it to retain moisture.

3.   **Manage Tangles**- Hair breaks and falls at a large rate when it is difficult to comb hair easily. One of the biggest contributors to hair breakage is hair tangles. Using Apple Cider Vinegar along the length of the hair keeps it well moisturized. As a result the surface of the hair also flattens out making it easy to detangle the hair. We will notice that with regular use it becomes easier to glide the comb down the length of the hair.

4.   **Treat Hair Loss**- When hair becomes more manageable and more conditioned it is less prone to breakage and damage. Most hair fall is caused by breakage while combing the hair. Using Apple Cider Vinegar reduces the

chances of hair fall due to tangled hair in addition to that the acidic properties Apple Cider Vinegar also cleans off the oil glands present below the hair follicle. This stimulates hair growth and makes your locks longer and thicker.

5.   **Cleansing of the Scalp**- Many of us ignore the importance of our scalp as a part of our hair treatment regimen. However besides regular shampooing and washing our hair requires additional care to ensure that the scalp is free from dry skin and dandruff. It is a good idea to apply a mixture of Apple Cider Vinegar and baking soda on the scalp for a thorough cleansing routine. Many people have found this combination so useful that they entirely replaced shampoos and other chemical based products with this natural and economic option.

6.   **Clarifying Treatment**- When we use chemically treated hair products there is always some residue even after thorough washing. Over a period of time these chemicals build up in the scalp and make our hair weak and brittle. It is necessary to ensure that the chemical build up is removed on a regular basis. Apple Cider Vinegar is a perfect product for this purpose. This is because it is strong enough to remove the chemical entirely but is also mild enough to ensure that the scalp is not stripped of its natural oils.

7.   **PH Balance**- In order to grow properly our hair requires a recommended PH level which lies in the range of 4.5 to 5.5. This means our hair is mildly acidic in nature and it requires a product that can maintain this acidity. The good news is that Apple Cider Vinegar has an acidity that is very similar to our hair. So it is recommended that you rinse your hair with Apple Cider Vinegar every time you shampoo it to make sure that the PH level is retained

8.   **Controlling Frizz-Frizzy** hair always looks unkempt and is also difficult to manage and often turns brittle if left untreated. Apple Cider Vinegar along with baking soda is a perfect frizz control treatment. This method ensures that the treatment reaches every strand of your hair. As a result all the strays are controlled and every strand of hair becomes shinier and easier to maintain. Of course it is also visually pleasing as the hair looks like it is in place and not just one big unmanageable bunch.

9.   **Treatment of Itchy and Dry Scalp**-Apple Cider Vinegar is known for its ability to fight bacteria and fungus. Often infections like certain strains of bacteria or virus make the scalp itchy, dry and flaky. In some severe conditions scabs are produced on the surface of the scalp. When these fall or are plucked they release pus that blocks the oil glands present

below the hair follicle. As a result the hair does not receive the nourishment that it requires. Consequently it becomes weak and dull.

10.   **Prevention of Split Ends**- Split Ends gives our hair the appearance of being very unmanageable and dull. It is also believed that split ends prevent hair growth and also lead to life less hair. Regularly rinsing your hair with Apple Cider Vinegar helps control this condition. In addition to that, your hair also gets a beautiful bounce. Since hair fall also reduces the volume increases automatically.

Apple Cider Vinegar is undoubtedly one of the best options for a good natural hair care treatment. It is available easily, is inexpensive and is also very easy to apply. It is no wonder that it finds a place in most folk remedies. You can also prepare your own Apple Cider Vinegar at home.

All you need to do is mix one part of warm water to one part of Apple Cider Vinegar. Make sure that the water you are using is filtered. After the regular shampooing regimen all you need to do is apply this homemade rinse. In case you think your hair needs more conditioning you may leave it on your hair for a couple of minutes before you rinse off with water. It is recommended that you use this hair care product at least once week for maximum results.

Apple Cider Vinegar for the Skin

Many adolescents and adults struggle with the problem of acne. Very few know that Apple Cider Vinegar is a very useful product to help take care of skin and get rid of acne breakouts forever. Of all the home care remedies that are recommended it has been observed that Apple Cider Vinegar is the most effective one. The question is how Apple Cider Vinegar aids the betterment of skin in comparison to other products.

Apple Cider Vinegar that has been made from organic apples and has been left unfiltered consists of a substance known as mother of vinegar. It is in this cloudy substance that several enzymes and minerals that are beneficial to the skin are found. Hence it is always recommended that you shake your bottle of Apple Cider Vinegar well every time you use it so that these enzymes are released into the liquid.

Apple Cider Vinegar has the same constituents as apples. One such component is malic acid which contributes largely to the skin care benefits of Apple Cider Vinegar. This component gives Apple Cider Vinegar its anti bacterial, anti fungal properties. This helps it prevent acne and skin infections and also combat common dermatological problems. One of the most contributing factors for acne is production of excessive oil in the glands present at the base of our skin. Apple Cider Vinegar is useful in removing this excess oil to ensure that these glands are not infected to create outburst and acne. The maintenance of PH balance of skin is another important function of Apple Cider Vinegar. It ensures that the oil secretion in the skin is normalized to make sure that it doesn't become too dry or too oily.

Apple Cider Vinegar also acts as a great exfoliating agent. You must have noticed that most commercial skin care products that are priced very high advertise the presence of alpha hydroxy acids in their preparation. However Apple Cider Vinegar forms a cheaper and a more effective alternative to these products. The role of alpha hydroxy acids is to remove the layer of dead skin cells to provide a healthier complexion also the layer of skin under the dead skin is a fresher and healthier one and this contributes to the youthful glow that Apple Cider Vinegar promises.

Age spots are another common dermatological problem that many women grapple with. It has been found that mixing Apple Cider Vinegar with fresh orange juice or even onion juice provides desirable results. All you need to do is apply this mixture over the age spots several times in a day. If your skin is sensitive this application may sting slightly. However there is no need to panic as it is not the side effect.

Apple Cider Vinegar is one of the only natural products that is effective in treating warts. A small ball of cotton wool soaked in Apple Cider Vinegar and pressed against the wart with a tape or band aid is the most effective remedy. You make keep this application on all day or you may just use overnight. It has been observed that warts clear up within a week. You must remember that the wart will turn completely black before it falls off. If you continue to use Apple Cider Vinegar even after the warts have gone you can be rest assured that they may not appear again.

Apple Cider Vinegar when consumed internally promotes healthy skin. This is mainly because it detoxifies the body and treats any condition related to digestion. Apple Cider Vinegar promotes better functioning of your liver. The main function healthy liver is to remove toxins from your body. Usually the liver is overworked because of poor digestion. This has an effect on your skin which is the first reflection of any toxic overload in the body.

For those who only believe in topical application of Apple Cider Vinegar you can create your own apple vinegar face wash at home. All you need to do is mix Apple Cider Vinegar with water in a 1:3 ratio. When you are accustomed to use Apple Cider Vinegar you can make this face wash more concentrated and bring up the ratio to 1:1.

To make sure that your skin is not over sensitive to Apple Cider Vinegar a patch test is always recommended. Apply a small amount to your elbow or any hidden part of your face. Allow this mixture to sit on your skin for an hour and look for any adverse reaction. If there is a problem you may use Apple Cider Vinegar in a much diluted form. Once you have become comfortable using Apple Cider Vinegar as a face-wash you can include it in your daily beauty regimen. To begin with wash your face with lukewarm water following that wipe your face with a cotton ball dipped in Apple Cider Vinegar. Cover the entire area including your neck. Make sure that all the strokes you use are upward and gentle.

You can use Apple Cider Vinegar to create deep core treatment packs that will remove any dirt and grime present in your face. A mixture of Apple Cider Vinegar, honey and fullers earth clay can be applied on the skin and left for 10 to 15 minutes. When you wash it off you will notice that your skin is supple and soft.

Many people have found useful skin remedies by simply replacing their usual toner with Apple Cider Vinegar. You can just use a mixture of Apple Cider Vinegar and water all over your skin. This ensures that your complexion is clear and all the freckles and age spots diminish. It also prevents accumulation of cellulite on your face.

Apple Cider Vinegar is also known for fighting signs of ageing. This is because it contains a large amount of Sulfur. Sulfur is useful in tightening the skin and also reducing the chances of fine lines and wrinkles. It is recommended that you apply Apple Cider Vinegar directly on your face each night and simply wash it off with water the next day.

Apple Cider Vinegar is also a powerful astringent. Therefore it is useful against any inflammation or redness that might be found on the skin. It is also effective against sunburns. All you need to do is apply a small amount of Apple Cider Vinegar on the affected area for immediate results.

The thumb rule to use Apple Cider Vinegar is that you must dilute it any time you feel a sting on your skin. This pinch or sting is only caused because your skin is sensitive and is not any side effect on using Apple Cider Vinegar.

Beauty Benefits of Coconut Oil

Coconut oil applications for the hair

Coconut oil is the most popular hair care remedy in the Asian subcontinent. It has been voted as the most beneficial natural oil in hair care. Even in its crudest form coconut oil is nothing but beneficial for the hair. The natural creamy texture of the coconut oil allows you to apply it in the scalp and along the length of the hair easily. There are also several odorless varieties that are available in the market. These varieties can be applied and left on the hair all day long for maximum positive results.

In many cultures, the application of coconut oil before washing the hair is mandatory. This adds luster to the hair and also helps bring back the natural texture of the hair. The application of coconut oil is also extremely therapeutic. It relieves stress and also keeps the scalp cool and rejuvenated with regular application.

Coconut oil is as good as, if not better, than the most popular salon treatment. This treatment can be practiced on your own in the comfort of your home. It is also available at the fraction of the cost, making it the most obvious choice for hair care. Coconut oil is useful for hair care because:

- **It prevents hair loss:** Coconut oil has been used as a hair fall remedy for several centuries. People who suffered from alarming rates of hair loss resorted to coconut oil as a recommended remedy. These individuals noticed the effects of using coconut oil within one month of regular use. Even the crown of the hair where hair re-growth is most difficult witnessed a significant increase in volume.

The hair care regiment was quite simple. It involved the application of two table spoons of coconut oil to the hair and scalp. After a gap of about 30 minutes, the oil can be washed off. This routine can be followed on a daily basis or at least once in two days for maximum benefits.

- **It conditions the hair:** Coconut oil is one of the best natural hair conditioners. it can also be treated as a leave in hair conditioner for best results. You may apply the non stick and the odorless variants of coconut oil that are available in the market and just allow your hair to soak it in. You can even try the wet towel method which is quite effective. All you need to do is apply a generous amount of coconut oil on your hair and scalp. Then, soak a thick towel in hot water and squeeze the excess water out. Wrap this towel around your hair and allow it to stay for a couple of minutes.

Coconut oil is great in retaining the moisture content of your hair. It reduces the number of stray hairs and is therefore effective in controlling the presence of frizz.

- **It promotes the growth of hair:** Coconut oil can be massaged to the scalp on a regular basis. On its own, coconut oil has the ability to relieve stress and soothe the muscles. The massage also stimulates circulation of blood to the roots of your hair. As a result, hair growth is promoted. With regular application, hair becomes thick and voluminous.

Coconut oil is also a great cleansing agent because of its antibacterial and antifungal properties. Therefore, applying coconut oil to your scalp also cleanses the oil secreting glands that are essential for hair growth. Once these glands are able to keep the scalp supple and moisturized, hair growth will increase.

- **It retains the protein content of the hair:** Our hair is made up of proteins, as we all know. In many cases, hair becomes brittle and undergoes a lot of breakage because of protein loss. Recently, a study was conducted by the Journal of cosmetic science to understand the benefits of different oils that are commonly used in hair regimens. This included sunflower oil and other mineral oils. The study revealed that only coconut oil was effective in reducing the loss of proteins from the hair. Both damaged and undamaged hair can be repaired and protected respectively when coconut oil is used as a grooming product before or after washing. This is because coconut oil is rich in medium chain fatty acids. These acids go deep into the shaft of the hair and ensure that there is no loss of proteins. As a result, hair begins to look smooth, silky and shiny with regular application of coconut oil.

- **It helps prevent dandruff:** The primary cause of dandruff is dry and flaky scalp. The scalp retains this condition only when the amount of natural oils produced by the glands present at the root of our hair is not good enough. These glands, known as sebaceous glands, often produce smaller amount s of natural oils when they are either blocked or infected. There are several kinds of yeast like fungus that live on the scalp. They mostly feed on the skin oils and are instrumental in yielding dandruff. Using coconut oil ensures that these kinds of microbes are permanently removed from the scalp to reduce the chances of dandruff.

The regular use of coconut oil ensures that the scalp is nourished. The antibacterial and antifungal properties of coconut oil ensure that there is no infection of the gland. Coconut oil is also a strong cleansing agent which is capable of removing all the dead skin and cells from the scalp. As a result, flaky skin can be prevented, and so can be dandruff.

The regular use of coconut oil gives you trade the shine and bounce that no other product is capable of giving. When you are too stressed out or even unwell, a good coconut oil massage has several positive results. The best part is that the routines that involve coconut oil are the simplest to practice. Since this oil is not too viscous, it is absorbed by the hair. In addition to that, it is also very easy to wash off as well.

Coconut oil for the skin

Coconut oil is one of the best skin care products. It has the ability to nourish skin and make it extremely soft and supple. The unique medium chain fatty acids that are present in coconut oil have great skin care properties. They act as anti fungal and anti bacterial agents and are perfect to help skin stay free from acne and outbursts.

In addition to that, medium chain fatty acids also have the ability to release antioxidants into the skin, leaving it fresh and glowing. Of course, coconut oil is one of the most medium chain fatty acid- rich components that is found in nature. As a result, it makes a great skin care regimen and is also food for your skin. The skin care benefits of coconut oil include:

- **Intense Moisturizing**

Using coconut oil that is cold pressed works really well on the skin. It serves as a multi vitamin source for the skin. Any good quality virgin coconut oil is perfect for your skin as in nourishes even the deeper layers of the skin. To moisturize the skin we can whip the coconut oil to give it an airy and creamy texture. This works as a great cold cream and moisturizer in the winter months.

- **Emollient to the skin**

The main constituent of coconut oil is the medium chain fatty acids. These packs seep into the skin and provide a very soothing and softening effect. They also help heal wounds that are caused by acne and pimples. Other cuts and boils that are formed on the skin also heal very quickly when coconut oil is applied. Any dryness or itchiness on the skin is soothed immediately after applying coconut oil. Therefore it is also been used as an effective treatment for conditions like dermatitis and psoriasis.

- **Nourishment for the skin**

The medium chain fatty acids that are present in coconut oil act as food for the skin. These fats can be absorbed by the skin to produce energy to give it a healthy and glowing effect. When nourishment is provided to the skin with coconut oil it also becomes self sufficient and is able to heal itself.

- **Antiseptic and Anti-microbial**

There is no drug that has been approved by the FDA which has both anti fungal and anti bacterial properties. Coconut oil is one such natural product which is able to provide our skin with this dual action. Applying coconut oil on skin on regular basis ensures that it is kept clean. All the microbes that are normally found on the skin are limited when coconut oil is applied. This ensures that skin infection that causes conditions like eczema and dermatitis are less common.

- **Natural treatment for acne**

Usually oily skin is considered to be the breeding grounds for microbes that cause acne. So coconut seems like a rather unconventional treatment for a condition which can be aggravated by all this. However the fats found in coconut oil have a very unique property. They are not thick and hence do not block the pores. On the other hand they act as very useful anti bacterial agents that can curb infections right at the onset. In order to treat acne apply a thin layer of coconut oil on your skin. Steam the surface of the skin and then gently wipe off the coconut oil. It is recommended that you keep coconut oil for no longer than 20 minutes on the skin. Any painful cut or wound caused by acne can be healed and soothed with coconut oil.

- **Powerful anti oxidant**

Most of the ageing and wrinkling is caused by the presence of free radicals in our skin. The only best way to combat this is by using substances that are rich in anti oxidants. Coconut oil is one of nature's best providers of anti oxidants. It consists of two important components called ferulic acid and p-coumaric acid. These two components are very useful in removing free radicals and hence slowing the ageing process. Any wrinkle that is already present on the skin is smoothened out when coconut oil is used on regular basis.

- **Younger looking skin**

In most cases skin begins to look dull and lifeless because of presence of a layer of dead skin. The skin that is present just below this layer is healthy, glowing and younger looking. Coconut oil acts as a great exfoliating agent and is useful in getting rid of all the dead cells on the skin to make it look healthy and supple.

- **Great Massage**

Coconut oil is the most commonly used massage oil. It is the texture and the component of this oil that makes it easy for the skin to absorb it. A good massage with coconut oil leaves the skin feeling soothed and relaxed. Regular massage with coconut oil also improves blood circulation to the skin and helps get rid of discoloration, dark circles and even darkened knees and elbows.

- **Great Deodorant**

Quite contrary to most of our beliefs sweat is actually odorless. The unpleasant smell that arises when we sweat is basically due to the action of bacteria and microbes that are present on our skin. The microbe killing property of the medium chain fatty acids found in coconut oil can actually help eliminate body odor.

This is because coconut oil does not allow bacteria to thrive and therefore allows sweat to retain its natural odorless form. Applying coconut oil in problem areas like the arm pits can actually reduce the problem of bad odor.

Applying coconut oil is recommended at least twice a week initially. In case there is any irritation on the skin it is recommended that you consult your doctor before continuing the use. However unless the oil that is used is impure and crude there should not be any adverse effect on your skin. The best thing about coconut oil is that it forms a very simple and economic option for your skin.

Chapter 5: Household Applications

Household Uses of Coconut Oil

Of course, the health benefits and the beauty benefits of coconut oil are known to us now. In addition to this, coconut oil can be used in our homes to take care of several painful chores. Some benefits of coconut oil include:

- **Cleaning leather:** Coconut oil is one of the best cleansers found in nature. In order to cleanse the leather furniture in your home, all you need to do is apply a small amount of coconut oil on cotton swab. Now run it in circles along the leather surface until it is absorbed by the surface completely.

- **Furniture polish:** Just as you would use coconut oil on leather, you can also use is to polish the furniture in your home. Coconut oil is great in removing dirt from the grains that are found in the wood. Natural oils like coconut oil are very useful in nourishing the wood. As a result, the longevity of your furniture increases. The use of coconut oil in varieties of wood like teak and rosewood helps maintain the natural shine of these kinds of woods.

- **Mosquito repellent:** The thought of going out after the dark is often quite unpleasant because of the insects and mosquitoes that will attack you the moment you step out. Of course there are several chemical products that are available in the market. However, these products may have more adverse effects on your skin that any insect bite. It is recommended that you make a spray using coconut oil and peppermint and use it on your skin every time you need head outdoors. This is a very effective insect repellent that has been used for decades.

- **Removal of residue:** Coconut oil, as mentioned before, is a great solvent. Usually, on all the furniture and new products that we bring into our home, the biggest problem is that of gum residue. No matter what soap or cleaning agent you use, getting rid of these residues seems impossible. In such cases, all you need to do is apply a thin layer of coconut oil over the residue. Allow it to soak for a few minutes. Then, use a rag to wipe the residue off. Coconut oil is gentle and will therefore work without spoiling the fabric or your furniture.

- **Lubricant:** In our homes, lubricants are always in demand. Whether it is fixing creaky hinges of the cupboards in your kitchen or bed room or just preventing the ceiling fan from making a rattle all night long, lubricants are extremely useful. One multipurpose and easily available lubricant is coconut oil. No matter what you need to lubricate you can use coconut oil. Several homes have replaced a common household lubricant called WD-40 with coconut oil. The mild properties of coconut oil are an important reason for this switch. You can be rest assured that your appliances and furniture will not be damaged.

- **Seasoning of Pans:** Before using pans for cooking, it is necessary to season them completely. This renders them non sticky and also ensures that the food is evenly cooked. Coconut oil is one if the best lubricating agents that you can use in pans. In addition to the fact that it seasons pans and maintains the material, coconut oil is also recommended because the nutritional benefits are passed on to the foods that are cooked in these pots and pans. All you need to do spray a layer of coconut oil on pans made of iron and also other kitchen appliances.

- **Cleaning the shower:** Shower scum is one of the most difficult things to get rid of. If you are using hard water in your house, the scum formed is a lot more stubborn and is harder to get rid of. In such cases, coconut oil acts as a very powerful cleansing agent. For best results, it is recommended that you use the coconut oil along with white vinegar. Just spray the mixture over the area that you want to clean. After sometime, just wipe it off with a rag. The tiles will sparkle and will look as good as new.

- **Detailing of the car:** Maintaining your car is a very difficult process. There are several cleaning agents that claim that they are useful in detailing your car. There is no doubt that these chemical based products are commonly used by car owners. However, they contain several chemicals that are not only harmful for the car but may also have harmful effects on people who are using the car regularly. Using coconut oil to detail your car is a great idea. All the dust and dirt from the nooks and crannies of your car can be removed completely. Coconut oil is also useful in keeping the interiors of your car cleaner for longer.

- **To clean mouth guards:** Mouth guards and retainers are most prone to bacterial and fungal growth. Keeping them clean is mandatory to ensure that there are no adverse health effects because of the use of these unclean retainers. Coconut oil has several antibacterial properties that can kill all the bacteria growing on these retainers or mouth guards. All you need to do is apply some coconut oil on the retainer and leave it all day. This will remove traces of any bacterial. Following this, you must rinse the retainer well before using it.

Coconut oil is undoubtedly one of the most versatile products of nature. Not only does it have several unimaginable health and beauty benefits, it is also useful around your home. So, if you are looking for a product that can promote complete personal and home care needs, all you need to do is buy yourself a bottle of coconut oil.

Household Uses of Apple Cider Vinegar

Apple vinegar is one of the most powerful cleansing agents found in nature. It is the strong acidic property of this substance that makes it extremely useful in household applications. Many homes prefer the use of apple cider vinegar over chemically available products as this is the healthiest and the most obvious choice for people who are worried about the health and well being of their family. The uses of Apple Cider Vinegar in a household include:

- **As a cleansing agent:** Apple Cider Vinegar is great for cleaning household appliances. All you need to do is mix a portion of apple cider vinegar with water and apply it on the area of you house or the appliance that you want to clean. The acidic property of Apple Cider Vinegar ensures that any scum or soap residue that is seen in appliances and in areas of the house such as the bathroom or the kitchen is removed almost instantly when it is applied. If the mildew, grime or scum in your shower area, the bathtub or even the tiles of your kitchen is bothering you, all you need to do is spray a generous amount of Apple Cider Vinegar and wipe it off after a while.

- **Remove oil from pots and pans:** The most common problem that we face with pots and pans is the accumulation of oil and even food stains over a period of time. This makes the utensils quite undesirable to look at. In such cases, all you need to do is apply a generous amount of Apple Cider Vinegar on the vessel. Following this, you must just rinse the utensils in hot water to make sure that all the stains are gone.

- **Cleaning Windows:** If you dread cleaning your windows because it is a time consuming process, it is recommended that you give Apple Cider Vinegar a shot. All you need to do is spray Apple Cider Vinegar on the window panes and wipe them completely clean. The stains, the grime and the dust are removed by the acidic nature of Apple Cider Vinegar, making your job a lot easier.

- **Removing stains for your carpet:** If you have pets at home, then the most common problem that you will face is that of stubborn stains of your carpet. Even marks like wine spills or even sauce stains can be extremely hard to get rid of. In such cases, using Apple Cider Vinegar can be of great help. All you need to do is mix equal portions of Apple Cider Vinegar and water. Run this mixture over the stain several times. When you are sure that the stain is gone completely, all you need to do is blot the excess liquid. Once your carpet is dry, you will see that the stain has vanished entirely.

- **Removing lime build up:** With the use of hard water comes one of the most difficult household problems- Lime build up. The areas that are most commonly affected are the shower enclosures and the tiles of your bathroom. The deposits leave the tiles looking old and lifeless. If you are looking for a quick remedy for this issue, I would suggest Apple Cider Vinegar as an effective measure.

- **Deodorizing your home:** Apple Cider Vinegar is useful in removing any undesirable smell from your household. If you find that a certain room in your house has a strong cigarette smell or any other strong odor, all you need to do is place a jar of apple cider vinegar in the room somewhere. Sometimes, even the garbage disposal develops a peculiar odor that can make its way to any corner of your home. In such cases all you need to do is pour a cup of Apple Cider Vinegar along with ice cubes into the garbage disposal.

- **Keeping ants away:** if your home is attacked and invaded by ants frequently, Apple Cider Vinegar might be the solution that you are looking for. All you need to do is spray a mixture of vinegar with an equal proportion of water. Make sure you cover all the entry points of these pests into your home. This includes the window sills, the door and any small hole of gap that the ants can make their way into your house through.

- **Prevent fading of clothes:** If you are worried about your clothes fading away in the sun, you can use Apple Cider Vinegar as a useful preventive measure. All you need to do is soak your clothes in water containing Apple Cider Vinegar before washing them. This way, even when they are dried in the sun, clothes will remain bright and will look new all the time.

- **Prevent formation of ice on your windshield:** if you are sick of waking up each morning and spending a lot of time defrosting your window shield, you might want to dig out the jar of Apple Cider Vinegar in your closet. To prevent the deposit of ice, all you need to do is pour two cups of Apple Cider Vinegar over the windshield and then rinse it off with a little water.

- **Removing Wall Paper:** If you are considering getting rid of the wallpaper in your home, you need not worry. It is not a very difficult process if you have Apple Cider Vinegar at home. All you need to do is make a mixture if hot water and apple cider vinegar in equal parts. Now rub this over the wallpaper that you want to remove. When the mixture is soaked in completely, the wall paper will begin to peel off on its own.

- **Flowers and Grass:** If you have unwanted weed growing in your bed of flowers and grass, all you need to do is pour Apple Cider Vinegar in the affected area directly to prevent further weed growth.

Apple Cider Vinegar has several other uses in a household. The bottom line is that the strong acidic property of Apple Cider Vinegar makes it a very powerful cleansing agent. It also makes it a disinfectant and a reliable deodorizer. You can choose to purchase Apple Cider Vinegar from the store or can even make it at home for the best results.

Chapter 6: Extracting ACV and coconut oil at home

Extracting Coconut Oil at Home

What is better than natural, virgin coconut oil? Coconut oil that is freshly extracted at home! Now, you might think that this elaborate industrial process cannot be carried out in your kitchen. However, quite contrary to what we expect, coconut oil can be extracted easily in your home. This product is not only 100% pure but also allows you to be sure of the ingredients that have been used to create it.

To begin with, you need two large coconuts that are completely ripe and mature. I recommend shaking the coconut, holding it close to your ears. If you are able to hear the rattle of the kernel, chances are that the coconut meat has turned into copra. On the other hand, if you are able to hear the sound of coconut water, get ready to prepare some exquisite coconut oil in your home.

Break the shell of the coconut and scrape the meat out using a knife and a spoon. Once you have all the shavings of the coconut meat, put them into a food processor and blend using cold water. Remove it only when you have a fine paste. The next step is to extract the coconut oil from this paste. In the industrial process you have huge mechanical presses to do the job. In your home, all you require is a cheese cloth or a flat juice strainer.

Pour the blended meat into the processor and squeeze with all your might. Of course, collect the extracts in a bowl. You will see that he extract resembles milk. It is a white viscous liquid that is known as coconut milk. The next step is to separate the contents of the milk to get your divine, fresh coconut oil.

Place the coconut oil on the stove and set the flame on low. Allow the coconut milk to simmer. After a few hours, you will see that all the cream has collected on the top. This is when you can turn the flame off and transfer the contents in to the refrigerator. Allow it to cool overnight. When you take it off the next morning, you will see that all the cream has solidified.

You can now slice the cream and scoop it out. Transfer this into another pot to prevent any mess. This cream needs to be heated on low flame for a couple of hours. Then you will see that the oil separates from the cream. All the other contents of the coconut cream will turn brown. The clear oil will be visible, separated from them.

Now, you need to scoop the oil and place it in a glass jar. Remember to stir the cream constantly when it has been placed on the stove. When you do this, the oil separates faster. It is a lot of hard work, no doubt. However, the oil that you are able to extract will smell divine. You can also simply try this process once to compare the quality of homemade coconut oil to the ones you buy in the store. The results will blow you away!

Making Apple Cider Vinegar at Home

For several years, people have resorted to simple fermentation techniques to produce wine in their homes. Now vinegar is just a fancy French word for "Sour wine". So, if you are able to make wine at home, you must definitely be able to make Apple Cider Vinegar at home. The process is slightly time-consuming. However, the results are extremely satisfactory and the actually method of producing Apple Cider Vinegar at home is not as hard as you think.

It is best recommended that you use organic apples to make your cider. Wash these apples (approximately 10 of them) and slice them into quarters. Let these slices rest at room temperature. As expected, they will turn brown. Take these browned apples in a glass jar and cover them with water. The level of water should be just enough to drown all the slices.

Now, take a cheese cloth and simply place it over the jar. You need not tie it or secure it as you need to allow oxygen to enter the apples that have been soaked in the water. Now, find a warm place in your home and just place the whole apparatus as it is. This jar must be allowed to rest for at least six months. Make sure that you stir it at least once a week.

After six months, take this jar down. You will notice the formation of a layer of scum at the surface of the jar. This is the result of the fermentation of the apples due to bacteria. The layer will almost look like bubbles that you see in a bucket of water when you throw in some soap and shake it.

The next step is to filter this liquid. Take a larger jar and place a cheese cloth over the jar containing the apples. This time, secure the cheesecloth tightly. Just tip the jar containing apples over the larger jar. The liquid will trickle through this into the second jar. Allow the entire liquid to be transferred into your larger jar.

Now, the new jar of liquid must be allowed to rest in a warm place. It should not be touched for at least four weeks. At the end of this long wait, you will have some beautiful amber colored apple cider vinegar that can be used for several home remedies.

The advantages of using homemade apple cider vinegar and coconut oil are many. Not only are they more effective in yielding results, they are also purer forms that reduce the risks of side effects. Since you are the one who made it, you can be sure of the hygiene and the cleanliness of the entire process.

Of course, they might test your patience the first few times. However, when you are able to see the health benefits and are able to experience the joy of creating these exotic ingredients in your kitchen, it will all be worth it!

Chapter 7: Best of Both Worlds

Here are some simple recipes that help you experience the benefits of Apple Cider Vinegar and coconut oil together. The soothing and relaxing property of coconut oil when mixed with the fierce acidic property of apple cider vinegar produces effects on your health and well being that are quite unimaginable:

Apple Cider Vinegar and Coconut Oil for lice

Lice can be very difficult to get rid of once they have made their way into the depths of your long locks. Especially when lice have started to lay eggs on the hair shaft, you can be assured that this is a rather severe problem that you need to take care of.

If you are in a dilemma about using the best products to eradicate lice while maintaining the luster and the shine of the hair, you can use the dual action of apple cider vinegar and coconut oil. To begin with, rinse the hair thoroughly with apple cider vinegar. If the lice infestation is too much, you can also leave the apple cider vinegar in for a few minutes. Allow it to dry up completely before you move on to the next step.

The next step is to massage the scalp and the hair with coconut oil. The entire volume of the hair must be covered with coconut oil to ensure optimum benefits. Cover the hair with a shower cap and just leave this mixture on for the whole day.

The mixture of Apple Cider Vinegar and coconut oil will smother the lice and kill them in a couple of hours. When you take the shower cap off, simply comb your hair to get rid of all the lice and eggs. Wash the hair thoroughly with your regular shampoo after this. This amazing hair mask not only ensures that your hair is free from lice; it also gives your hair shine and volume. So, while you are getting a full power lice treatment, you are also getting a great hair nourishing treatment.

Oil Cleansing for your Skin

There is no better remedy for your skin than a thorough oil cleansing regimen. This is a simple procedure that you can try in the comfort of your home. The first step is to prepare the mask for your face. For this, mix equal parts of honey and coconut oil. Massage it on the skin and allow it to be absorbed by your skin for a few minutes. When you feel like the pack is drying up, you can wash the pack off. Mixing grape seed oil or castor oil once in a while is also a great idea.

Now, you can finish off this treatment with a round of apple cider vinegar toner. Not only does this get rid of spots and coloration on the skin, it also acts like an astringent. So, if any wounds from acne and outbursts have been left behind, apple cider vinegar ensures that it is removed completely. So, this interesting skin care regimen gives your skin wholesome nourishment and also necessary antibacterial and antifungal treatment to keep it fresh and free from any infection.

There are other ways in which you can combine apple cider vinegar and coconut oil in your daily routine. You may simply consume a spoonful of each before your meals. This helps cleanse your system from the inside and makes you feel healthier. Both these products will help maintain your blood sugar level, cholesterol and blood pressure. They are powerful antioxidants that will help eliminate all the unwanted debris from you cells.

The result is that you will feel energized and fit. The positive effects of Apple Cider Vinegar and Coconut oil will reflect on your skin. You will see that it will have a gentle glow all the time, with a complexion to die for.

Chapter 8: Celeb Talk

Celebrity Secrets

When you think of skin care routines or general skin and health care, what is your standard to compare the results? Let's be honest, we always peep into magazines with gorgeous pictures and hope that our beauty and well being choices yield the same results. The good news is that apple cider vinegar and coconut oil are capable of just that!

Apple Cider Vinegar and Coconut oil have been testified by many Hollywood celebrities and sports stars as the secret to their well being. So, if you want to indulge like a celebrity, these two magic ingredients are perfect for you. Of course, one might also get a little cynical and wonder how these regular, everyday products could possibly interest celebrities who spend millions of dollars on their hair and skin care. Well, the best thing to do is to hear it from the horse's mouth. During my research, even I was taken aback to see how diligently most of my favorite celebs included my two favorite indulgences in their everyday life.

To begin with, the diva herself, Angelina Jolie, makes it a point to include virgin coconut oil in her breakfast along with a handful of cereal. This habit, she claims, allows her to manage her food consumption and prevent overeating.

And, guess who was spotted with a cart full of coconut oil? TV's own Rachael, Jennifer Aniston. She was an ardent follower of the coconut diet and vouched that it was effective in helping her lose weight and even keep metabolism high.

The gorgeous Miranda Kerr recently stated that she would not even go a single day without coconut oil. She consumes at least four spoons of coconut oil everyday and makes it a point to include it in her diet in the form of salads and even in her green tea. She has been using coconut oil as a beauty and health treatment since she was only 14 years old. This routine even helped her stay in shape after the birth of her first child, most renowned health experts believe.

If you ever wondered how Kourtney Kardashian manages to keep her black locks lustrous and thick, the answer is coconut oil. A celebrity fashion and lifestyle website stated that Kourtney's monthly hair regimen includes coconut oil, avocados, castor oil and eggs.

Oscar winning actress Gwyneth Paltrow, who was recently voted as the most beautiful woman on the planet, revealed a rather simple beauty treatment. Paltrow indulges in a detoxifying bath with Epsom salts. These salts help in exfoliating her skin and revive her muscles. To complete her routine, she uses virgin coconut oil as a moisturizer. This simple routine, according to her, helps keep her skin free from bumps and pimples and also keeps it stimulated at all times for the natural glow.

Some celebrities like Gisele Bundchen have gone the extra mile to take on infuriated dermatologists to promote a healthy and natural beauty product that they believe in. This Brazilian beauty recently released an organic skin care line that contains coconut oil as the primary ingredient. She stated that sunscreens are 'poisons' and that she would choose the humble coconut extract over any other sun blocking chemical. This did not put her in the 'favorite list' among dermatologists but it sure earned her skin care line a special place in the market.

Fitness guru Jillian Michaels stated that coconut oil is the best way to aid the immune system. Even in her book, "Master your Metabolism", she provides recipes in which coconut oil forms the main ingredient.

The one woman who personifies the meaning of the "ideal woman" for every man alive on this planet, Megan Fox is also quite simple in her ways. She ensures that she consumes a spoon of apple cider vinegar before each meal. This helps her maintain her perfect shape and her gorgeous skin and hair.

Scarlett Johansson who must keep her skin completely flawless being the face of Dolce and Gabanna also uses this common product. She vouches that this helps her maintain her gorgeous porcelain complexion and ensures that she is always camera ready. In a recent chat, Johansson said, "If your skin is problematic or you're having a lot of breakouts, it's really healing. It's a little bit stinky but if you're not sleeping over at your boyfriend's, it's really effective!"

She prefers the use of this simple organic product in comparison to chemical methods recommended by most dermatologists. She also states the benefits of Apple Cider Vinegar on the skin when it is simply used as a toner or a face wash. When it comes from a woman who is known across the globe for the healthy glow on her skin, we cannot help but take this suggestion seriously.

Another gorgeous lady who believes in gulping a spoonful of apple cider vinegar before every meal is Heidi Klum. This super model mixes apple cider vinegar with a glass of water and consumes it before every meal. Apple cider vinegar, she says, is so useful in curbing her hunger pangs that even a mere sniff is good enough to do the trick. It is a great detoxifying agent, she states, as the acidic property works beautifully to get rid of extra fats. Heidi Klum also sympathizes with individuals who are unable to consume Apple Cider Vinegar as it is quite unpalatable. To them, she suggests mixing apple cider vinegar with natural sweeteners like stevia. Of course, using sugar is out of question as it defeats the purpose of a natural, detoxifying dietary supplement.

This list contains just a handful of celebs and big names who believe in turning to natural remedies for their well being. The reason I included this section is that most of us compare ourselves to the people and the faces that we see regularly. When these individuals are able to maintain such desirable features with these simple and common remedies, so can we. It does not take millions of dollars to get beautiful skin, hair and a healthy body. All you need is the willingness to commit to a certain natural remedy and continue if patiently till you have the desired results.

Chapter 9: Precautions

Apple Cider Vinegar and coconut oil are undoubtedly some of the best products when it comes to healing various ailments. However we must ensure that these products are also consumed in recommended amounts. Usually they do not cause any harmful side effects or health problems. However too much of any good thin g can be disastrous. This is true for Apple Cider Vinegar and coconut oil as well.

Possible side effects of Apple Cider Vinegar

Whether consumed in the liquid or tablet form Apple Cider Vinegar is great for treating many health conditions. However you must always remember that Apple Cider Vinegar is highly acidic in nature. While controlled intake has PH balancing effects, too much consumption can imbalance the state of homeostasis in our body. Some harmful effects that your should watch out for are:

- Reduced potassium levels-The acetic acid content of Apple Cider Vinegar causes potassium deficiency which in turn leads to brittle and softer bones

- Digestive issues-No doubt Apple Cider Vinegar is a great remedy for acid reflux. However consuming too much causes diarrhea, heartburn and indigestion.

- Interactions with other medication

  If you currently taking insulin, laxatives or any such you must consult your doctor before of consuming Apple Cider Vinegar. This is because Apple Cider Vinegar may react with these medicines to have harmful effects on the body.

- Damaged tooth enamel

  Apple Cider Vinegar is high in its acidity. Therefore you must never consume it directly. It is best that you use a straw or opt for much diluted versions to maintain the enamel of the teeth. Prolonged exposure to Apple Cider Vinegar can make the enamel weak and yellowish in appearance. You may also immediately brush your teeth immediately after consuming this variety of to reduce damage.

Adverse effects of coconut oil

Coconut oil is one of the safest foods that you can consume. There have been very few cases of health adversities that have been reported. Only if you have certain food allergies will coconut oil harm you. So to make sure that it does not have any ill effects on your health it is best that you test on yourself before you consume it internally or externally. To do this, just rub a bit of coconut oil on your skin and leave for a day. If the skin is swollen or itchy, you have an allergy. In such cases you should consult your doctor or simply avoid coconut oil altogether. In worst cases of coconut oil allergies neurological damage and brain damage is also possible. So always con duct a test if you are new to coconut oil.

I have included this chapter in this book not to scare you or make you think twice about these amazing super foods. However any home remedy must practiced with great precaution. After all there is no way we can control how our body will react to different substances. So staying safe is the first step to staying healthy.

Chapter 10: Why Choose Organic Versions?

We have all heard of innumerable benefits of using organic products. These products are known for their natural properties. Basically, organic products are those which have not undergone any chemical processing. Even the raw materials that form the source of these products are grown using natural manures and methods.

With apple cider vinegar and coconut oil provide maximum benefits when they are used in their natural form. Only in the unprocessed forms of these products are all the useful nutrients present. For instance, in the organic form of apple vinegar a substance called "mother of vinegar" is present. This stringy layer consists of all the natural enzymes produced by the fermenting bacteria. These enzymes are very useful and form the basis

These enzymes are very useful and form the basis of all the health benefits of Apple Cider Vinegar. The process version is no doubt clear and more pleasant looking. However the nutritional benefits and other health benefits of this form of Apple Cider Vinegar are fewer.

Even in case of coconut oil it is recommended that we only opt for virgin coconut oil which the purest and most natural form available. Undoubtedly colder countries may opt for the versions like liquid coconut oil in order to ensure that it doesn't harden in cold conditions. This variety of coconut is treated heavily and is stripped of the fatty acids which form the basis of the healing abilities of coconut oil.

There have been several debates about the safety and advantages of using organic products. However research today shows that we have no other choice but to go the organic way. In process foods and natural products several chemicals are used which render these otherwise useful products quite harmful. For instance processed Apple Cider Vinegar or coconut oil can cause a lot of irritation and discomfort when used regularly. The organic products, on the other hand, are so safe that they can even be recommended for children.

Using Organic products can also be your way of contributing to the environment. Since these foods are grown without chemicals that are harmful to the environment they ensure that our planet does not deteriorate further. Using organic manures and pesticides make the soil richer. These plants require lesser water and hence play a pivotal role in water conservation.

Organic foods are best for consumption. These foods retain all the natural flavors that are most often missing in the processed versions. Obviously these foods taste better. Research shows that Apple Cider Vinegar and coconut oil have maximum mineral salts in their organic forms. As a result the health benefits of these products are also greater.

I personally recommend the use of organic products if you have children and pets at home you might want to switch to an organic way of life altogether. So in case these foods are accidentally consumed by them there are no adverse effects on their health. I have tried organic Apple Cider Vinegar and coconut oil and seen amazing results.

Conclusion

Thank you again for downloading this book!

I hope this book was able to help you to make use of these useful products that you will find sitting somewhere in your closet. I personally believe that the best and the most effective solutions to all our health issues are hidden somewhere in the depths of the kitchen.

Of course, I do not discourage the need to consult your doctor once in a while especially when symptoms fail to get suppressed. However, natural products like apple cider vinegar and coconut oil are the best precautionary measures that you can take against possible health issues.

The next step is to make these products a part of your daily routine. Since they also find applications in your household chores, I can assure you that they will become your most prized possessions over time. Of course, including them in your health regimen will take a bit of conscious effort in the beginning.

However, when you see the results, you will never forget your regular coconut oil and apple cider vinegar regime. Be prepared for loads of compliments from your friends and family. Also, you will find it amusing when they are unable to believe that something this simple can cause such dramatic effects. I have been there and it feels rather good.

Preview Of 'Digestive Health And Wellness

Chapter 1 A Holistic View on the Body

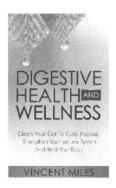

It is essential to clarify that a healthy gut is not only about assuring a fast digestion and having a good metabolism. True, keeping your gut clean will definitely result in the improvement of this part of your organism, but this is only one drop in the sea of overall effects that such a program will have.

A clean gut will improve both your physical and your mental state, since you will feel fresher and stronger. Weight loss is another significant result of maintaining an effective digestion through eating healthy. Your overall energy levels will change and psychologically you'll find you have a more vibrant state of mind, you feel much lighter in your body movements, you enjoy better concentration capacity, and a visible energy boost that will give you the strength you need in your daily activities.

Dr. Eva Cwynar, author of *The Fatigue Solution*, has already emphasized the role played by the digestive track in improving your general energy levels and performance. She recommends eating a lot of proteins in the morning, having small meals every 3-4 hours, and picking up mostly fresh fruit and vegetables, nuts and cereals as well as cheese and meat for your diet. In her opinion, all this will lead to a much better mood and overall capacity of your organism, as you'll be eating for energy, not for calories.

Dr. Alejandro Junger in his famous book *Clean Gut* goes even further and explains his belief that a dirty gut is at the root of all our health problems, even though we may not know it or we may only notice one link in the whole chain (a surface one), only one aspect in the overall dynamics of reactions that take place in our body. He considers the gut to be at the root of all disease if our digestion is left unchecked. It is wide known that severe diseases such as cancer, diabetes, autoimmune diseases, and even heart disease can be traced back to gut disorders. However what many of us may not be aware of is that even lighter forms of illness such as mood swings, constipation, fatigue, eczema, or low libido are caused by a less than perfect functioning of our digestive system ... at least to a certain extent. Of course there are myriad other disease causes, just as numerous as the sources of toxins we're exposed to nowadays! Aging is also a natural course and it is true that our body defenses weaken as time goes by. Naturally you would hardly think your libido is affected by the food you eat when you're over 50 and you don't feel as young and bouncy as you once did. Maybe you don't, but you can try to feel livelier and a healthy diet is one of the recommendable ways to go. A healthy gut is one of your main weapons in trying to slow down or attenuate the effects of aging. You will certainly not find any ambrosia or elixir for eternal life, but you can help your body stay young, more energetic and healthier for a longer while.

Did you know that, more or less literally, about two thirds of your immune system is in your gut? Your gut is like an ecosystem, with its varied flora of bacteria that help you process food you ingest, regulate digestion and hormones, excrete toxins, and produce vitamins or other compounds. Nature works according to an inner logic that is obviously extremely operative and simultaneously so discrete, that we can barely grasp it under normal circumstances. When something goes out of balance, we become aware of dysfunction. However more often than not it's hard to acknowledge that it may very well be something unwillingly provoked by ourselves through our eating habits and carelessness towards our organism. If the natural order in that ecosystem runs out of balance, the whole organism is likely to suffer and this in turn will have disruptive effects on your performance as an individual in many respects.

Picture a diaphanous convoluted chord in your body. That is the brain-gut connection. It's not immediately evident, because we learned to separate and evaluate the functions in our organism according to different systems whose activity appears quite independent. In reality our body works in concordance with an ingenious mechanism whose main force resembles electric current. When there's an energetic deficit due to disease or disorder in your gut, the flow to and in your brain will also be affected. Anatomically speaking, this connection between the gut and the brain explains why you can feel nausea or indigestion after you take antidepressants, why you can get depressive or get headache if you have bad digestion, why you either overeat, or you can't eat at all when you feel anxious, stressed out, sad, or terribly preoccupied with some problem. Even the butterflies in your stomach when you are in love or infatuated reflect this deep organic connection that we usually ignore. When you have to speak in public or to go on stage, why do you think you feel something shivering at the level of your gut, too? Because of this intrinsic connection between these two areas of your organism; sensitivity in one place reverberates in the other.

The bottom line is that some disease causes are easier to control and this is definitely the case when it comes to the health of our gut. Moreover, just as we should adopt a holistic take on your health; it's much better if we think long-term. When it comes to food, it's is without any doubt not easy to think of staying healthy ten years from now when you have a steaming steak in front of you or when your friend invites you to a cruelly tempting Pizza alla Diavola. Yes, you may feel you have to grab that hamburger in your break from work and get back to something serious fast. But as mature beings, if we can create some order in our lives, why not do it? It takes a great deal of determination and force of will, that's for sure. We also have to be very aware of the actual consequences of our impulsive eating: when we yield to a savory temptation, it's not only about feeling a bit bloated for the rest of the day or 'gaining' a pound or two. It's actually about making a decision about how much health you allow yourself to have in the future and even long you want the rest of your life to be. In other words, our diet is also about treasuring our bodies and about practicing love for ourselves.

Check Out My Other Books

Below you'll find some of my other books that are popular on Amazon and Kindle as well. Alternatively, you can visit my author page on Amazon to see other work done by me.

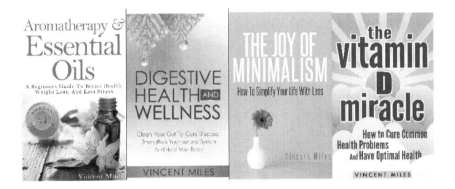

12729776R00059

Printed in Poland
by Amazon Fulfillment
Poland Sp. z o.o., Wrocław